YOUR KNOWLEDGE HAS VALUE

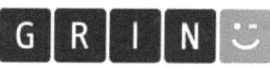

Bibliographic information published by the German National Library:

The German National Library lists this publication in the National Bibliography; detailed bibliographic data are available on the Internet at http://dnb.dnb.de .

Imprint:

Copyright © 2017 GRIN Verlag, Open Publishing GmbH
Print and binding: Books on Demand GmbH, Norderstedt Germany
ISBN: 9783668608566

This book at GRIN:

https://www.grin.com/document/385887

Patrick Kimuyu

Education Program for Breast Cancer Prevention in Women

GRIN Publishing

GRIN - Your knowledge has value

Since its foundation in 1998, GRIN has specialized in publishing academic texts by students, college teachers and other academics as e-book and printed book. The website www.grin.com is an ideal platform for presenting term papers, final papers, scientific essays, dissertations and specialist books.

Visit us on the internet:

http://www.grin.com/

http://www.facebook.com/grincom

http://www.twitter.com/grin_com

Education Program for Breast Cancer Prevention in Women

Name: Patrick Kimuyu

Abstract

A condition that affects women throughout all communities, breast cancer is a form of malignancy that affects the cells of the breast tissue. When diagnosed, this condition can result in aggressive treatment modalities including chemotherapy and breast mastectomy. In effort to decrease the diagnosis of breast cancer in women, adequate preventative methods are needed to assist the female population in decreasing the likelihood of disease. This paper offers women and Advanced Practice Nurses an educational program grounded in review of evidence-based research and guidelines that will assist in providing female patients with screening methods to detect breast cancer and modifiable risk factors that will assist in decreasing the likelihood of disease.

Table of Content

INTRODUCTION

A form of malignancy that affects the cells of the breast, breast cancer is diagnosed in one of eight women during their lifetime (Fogel & Woods, 2008). Breast cancer is a serious condition that reaches the lives of all members of the female population as up to 85% of women with newly diagnosed breast cancer do not have a family history of the condition (Buttaro et al., 2013). Women of all ages and ethnicities are being diagnosed with breast cancer with many of them unaware and uneducated concerning the prevention methods and lifestyle modifications that assist in decreasing the chance of developing the condition. Nurse practitioners play a crucial role in breast cancer prevention in women. As Advanced Practice Nurses continue to become an increased and strong presence in primary care provision for the population, they are able to provide teaching and education to women regarding their health and wellness and the prevention of breast cancer. The purpose of this paper is to provide an educational program for breast cancer prevention in women grounded in evidence-based research and guidelines concerning women's health. This educational program will assist practitioners in educating the target population of women in identifying, understanding and practicing the necessary interventions for breast cancer prevention. By utilizing this educational tool, Advanced Practices Nurses will be able to ensure successful breast cancer prevention in their female patients. Effective breast cancer prevention will be achieved by educating and encouraging women to complete important screenings such as BRCA testing and mammography, addressing modifiable risk factors such as obesity, alcohol and tobacco use and implementing interventions such as exercise and healthy eating.

LITERATURE REVIEW

In effort to develop this educational tool, a review of the literature was conducted to examine the different barriers faced by women to obtaining the necessary preventative screenings towards breast cancer prevention. These preventative methods include provider education, breast self-exams and mammography. This review of 15 research studies examines the level of knowledge of practitioners and patients as well as factors affecting decision making in breast cancer prevention. These studies were obtained using the CINAHL Plus nursing database where a large number of current Advanced Practice Nursing research articles are catalogued.

As medical providers play a crucial role in increasing women's awareness and understanding concerning breast cancer prevention, it is important to ensure that the knowledge level of these practitioners facilitates client education. An outcome analysis study by Edwards and Seibert sought to examine why nurse practitioners (NPs) fail to provide breast cancer risk assessment (BrCRA) to their clients (Edwards & Seibert, 2010). Thirty five nurse practitioners participated in this pretest-posttest study where the effectiveness of a BrCRA education program was conducted (Edwards & Seibert, 2010). The study found that the implementation of a BrCRA education program considerably increased nurse practitioners knowledge in assessing breast cancer risk thus demonstrating that appropriate counseling and education of NPs can assist in reducing women's risk of developing breast cancer (Edwards & Seibert, 2010).

Another study conducted by Edwards and colleagues examined nurse practitioners' knowledge and perceived comfort level in providing breast cancer risk assessment in the clinical setting (Edwards et al., 2009). This descriptive study surveyed 147 nurse practitioners at a national NP conference and found that assessing women's risk for the development of breast cancer is important in providing preventative strategies in breast cancer (Edwards et al., 2009). A statistically significant positive correlation was observed (0.39) between nurse practitioners' knowledge and comfort level in performing breast cancer risk assessment ($p < 0.001$) (Edwards et al., 2009). This study provides support for the continuous education of nurse practitioners concerning risk assessment of breast cancer and the ability to increase provider comfort level and thus assist in breast cancer prevention.

Bernard and colleagues surveyed 1,111 physicians registered with the American Medical Association with the purpose of describing practicing characteristics in reference to breast and cervical cancer early detection (Benard et al., 2011). The study found that use of screening methods was higher with physicians for whom beliefs in screening recommendations were integrated into their practices (Benard et al., 2011). Study results also suggest a correlation between use of regular screening methods and provider education regarding national guidelines and recommendations (Benard et al., 2011).

In addition to provider knowledge and practice, patient education and understanding plays a crucial role in breast cancer prevention. A cross-sectional study by Barghouti and colleagues utilized a questionnaire submitted to 602 female patients with the purpose of assessing knowledge and attitudes of women attending family practice clinics towards screening methods of breast cancer (Barghouti et al., 2012). The study found that women who had a higher knowledge score reported more breast self-exam (BSE) practices. Furthermore, the knowledge score was also a positive predictor of clinical breast-exams and obtaining mammograms (Barghouti et al., 2012).

Educational programs conducted throughout communities for female patients were also found to assist in increasing breast cancer prevention knowledge. Yi and Park conducted a pretest posttest study where a 60 minute educational program on breast cancer prevention methods was provided to twenty two women ages twenty to forty (Yi & Park, 2012). The study found that the scores on knowledge, skills, performance and self-efficacy before breast health education were significantly increased after 1 month and 3 months post-education thus demonstrating that providing women with breast health education programs including breast cancer prevention methods can significantly impact screening practices among women (Yi & Park, 2012).

Shalini and colleagues conducted a pretest posttest study among forty college women ages 18-19 with the purpose of assessing the level of knowledge of college female students on BSE (Shalini, Varghese & Nayak, 2011). The study included a 3 part questionnaire which consisted of demographics, BSE knowledge assessment and a teaching program (Shalini, Varghese & Nayak, 2011). The study found on the pretest that the majority of students did have an average level of BSE and that the teaching program is a useful and viable tool for breast self-examination awareness among young women (Shalini, Varghese & Nayak, 2011).

A study by Ozanne and colleagues sought to investigate decision making among women at high risk for breast cancer including preventative measures, understanding of disease as well as physician understanding of these factors. One hundred and forty-six women participated in a prospective interview and survey study. Results showed that physicians overestimated the decrease in perceived risk resulting from patient counseling ($p < 0.001$). In addition, women at high risk were found to overestimate their risk of disease thus showing the importance of knowledge and education of breast cancer prevention for both patients and providers.

Factors that assist in decreasing and assessing breast cancer risk in women were also reviewed in the literature. These factors include physical activity, mother-daughter relationship and mammography adherence. Ratnasinghe and colleagues examined the association between physical activity and breast cancer risk among 1,463 cancer cases and 4,862 controls in a multinational study (Ratnasinghe et al., 2010). Participants were asked how many times and for how long they exercised or engaged in vigorous physical labor a week (Ratnasinghe et al., 2010). The study found that the amount of time spent in physical activity a week was significantly associated with reduced risk. Study results also show that physical activity may reduce breast cancer risk regardless of race, weight or family history of breast cancer (Ratnasinghe et al., 2010).

Mother-daughter relationships have also been found to impact breast cancer prevention. A study by Sinicrope and colleagues sought to examine the degree to which mothers reported providing advice on breast cancer prevention to their daughters (Sinicrope et al., 2008). A questionnaire was mailed to 1,773 women and asked whether or not they had provided advice to their daughters on what they should do to prevent breast cancer (Sinicrope et al., 2008). The study found that breast cancer prevention behaviors were associated with providing advice (Sinicrope et al., 2008). Thus by increasing the level of knowledge and education to women and mothers on breast cancer prevention, daughters will benefit from the teaching and understand the importance of preventative methods.

Mammography adherence was also examined among women in a study by Watson-Johnson and colleagues. A focus group study was conducted to explore reasons why women who were previously adherent to regular mammography no longer were screened (Watson-Johnson et al., 2011). 20 focus groups were conducted with 128 women with discussion topics including mammography experience, perception of breast cancer risk and barriers to mammography (Watson-Johnson et al., 2011). The study found that major barriers to routine mammography exist including concerns about test efficacy, personal concerns about the procedure, access to screening services and psychosocial issues (Watson-Johnson et al., 2011). This study shows the importance of mammography education and access to care for women throughout communities.

In addition to adherence, several culturally-based barriers were identified in research studies conducted on breast cancer prevention. Kobetz and colleagues examined the barriers that exist in breast cancer screenings among Haitian women in Little Haiti, Miami (Kobetz et al., 2010). The study, which interviewed 15 women, found that 3 core categorical barriers exist to breast cancer prevention adherence: structural, psychological and socio-cultural (Kobetz et al., 2010). Furthermore, Mughivi and colleagues conducted a study that examined 200 rural women's knowledge of breast cancer prevention and found that rural women were unable to take responsibility for their breast health due to lack of knowledge (Mugivhi, Maree & Wright, 2009). Nuno and colleagues reached a similar conclusion when they examined breast cancer screening utilization among 504 Hispanic women living near the United States-Mexico border (Nuno et al., 2011). Their study found that women whose knowledge level of screening methods were higher, were more likely to obtain a mammogram and follow provider recommendations in comparison to women who lacked knowledge (Nuno et al., 2011). These studies show that additional education concerning breast cancer prevention is needed in effort to reach women from different cultural and societal backgrounds.

Specific sub-groups within the female population were also examined in the literature including lesbian women and women with intellectual disabilities. Hart and colleagues conducted a study that sought to examine the predictors of breast cancer screening in 150 self-identified lesbian/bisexual women as well as 400 heterosexual women (Hart & Bowen, 2009). The study found that there was a significantly positive relationship between sexual orientation and the intention to obtain a clinical breast exam and mammography (Hart & Bowen, 2009). Heterosexual women were more likely to obtain mammography whereas lesbian women felt embarrassed and procrastinated in obtaining the screening (Hart & Bowen, 2009).

Truesdale-Kennedy and colleagues also sought to examine breast cancer prevention beliefs among a specific group of women (Truesdale-Kennedy, Taggart & McIlfatrick, 2011). Their study examined 19 women with intellectual disabilities and their experiences with breast mammography (Truesdale-Kennedy, Taggart & McIlfatrick, 2011). Study results found participants to have several barriers to obtaining mammography including lack of information, embarrassment, fear and anxiety (Truesdale-Kennedy, Taggart & McIlfatrick, 2011). In effort to support these sub-groups within the female population, better education is needed for both women and providers in the provision of breast cancer screenings.

In conducting this review of literature, several factors were found to impact breast cancer prevention practices for both women and healthcare providers. Although several barriers were identified as affecting prevention adherence for women, the level of knowledge, attitude and understanding of breast cancer risks were found to be major factors that either prevented or assisted women in seeking care for breast cancer prevention. A summary table of the literature review is provided in Appendix A where the 15 research studies are synthesized and succinctly presented.

THEORETICAL FRAMEWORK

In addition to conducting a literature review, a nursing theory is utilized in effort to develop this educational tool grounded in research and theoretical principles. Dorothea Orem's *Self-Care Theory* is fitting for this project as it provides the necessary support to assist each individual woman in taking care and responsibility for their wellbeing (Orem, 1991).

8

Several philosophies in Orem's Theory apply to helping breast cancer prevention in women. Orem believed that people are distinct individuals and that people should be self-reliant and responsible for their own care and others in their family needing care (Orem, 1991).Furthermore, Orem found that a person's knowledge of potential health problems is necessary for promoting self-care behavior (Orem, 1991). Thus the more knowledge and understanding an individual has about potential health problems, the more likely they are to try to prevent or seek treatment for that problem.

As a nursing theorist, Dorothea Orem examined concepts in her theory that included nursing, health, the environment, human beings and nursing therapeutics (Orem, 1991). Orem's theory is grounded in 3 parts: the Theory of Self Care where the individual initiates activities and practices necessary to maintain life, health and well-being (Orem, 1991). Second, the Theory of Self Care Deficit where the need for nursing is identified and third, the Theory of Nursing Systems which describes how the patient self-care needs will be met (Orem, 1991). Orem's Self-Care theory also takes into consideration the level of social and interpersonal skills of both patient and care provider (Orem, 1991).

Several reasons make this nursing theory fitting to developing this educational tool. Orem's understanding that each person is an individual with their own needs and own way of learning is crucial to facilitating communication with women about breast cancer prevention (Orem, 1971). In addition, understanding that a person's knowledge of potential health problems dictates their behavior assists providers in focusing on education and creating a sense of self-care empowerment for women. Furthermore, identifying that care providers and patients each have a level of social or interpersonal skills makes it crucial to instill confidence not only in women about their care but providers as well regarding the care they provide.

For better self-care, providers must develop a patience and openness that welcomes women of all ages, race or socio-economic background. As Orem stated, the education and care provided must be grounded in care and understanding that each individual presents with their own level of understanding and of comfort concerning breast cancer prevention methods. Following Dorothea Orem's Self-Care Theory for breast cancer prevention in women will assist in creating an educational tool that can be used and understood by both patients and providers.

STANDARDS OF PRACTICE/PRACTICE GUIDELINES

Standards of practice exist that provide guidelines to providers in understanding breast cancer prevention methods. According to the American Cancer Society (ACS), early detection and screening is the best way to prevent breast cancer in women (American Cancer Society, 2012). Current ACS guidelines state that women age 40 and older should have a mammogram every year and should continue to do so as long as they are in good health. In addition, ACS guidelines state that women in their 20s and 30s should have a clinical breast exam as part of regular health exams by their providers preferably every 3 years (American Cancer Society, 2012). Starting at age 40, women should have a clinical breast exam by a medical provider every year although most providers include breast exams early on with well-woman exams for women who are sexually active (American Cancer Society, 2012).

The American Cancer Society also states that breast self-examination is an option for women starting in their 20s. The ACS recommends that women should be informed concerning benefits and limitations of breast-self exams and should immediately report any breast changes to their health professionals (American Cancer Society, 2012). Additionally, women at high risk should get an MRI (magnetic resonance imaging) and a mammogram every year. Women at moderately increased risk should speak to their healthcare providers concerning the benefits and limitations of yearly MRIs.

Further screenings recommended by the ACS include the BRCA and Brevagen testing (American Cancer Society, 2012). The BRCA test screens for breast cancer percentage risk in women with a high risk of breast cancer from a first degree relative such as a mother, sister or daughter and can be done at any age. Brevagen testing screens for breast cancer in women beginning age 35 with no significant risk factors for breast cancer but enables women to know their 5 year and their lifetime risk of developing breast cancer (American Cancer Society, 2012).

Lifestyle changes and modifications are also recommended to women of all race and ages as a simple but effective way to prevent breast cancer. These changes include consuming a healthy diet, exercising regularly and keeping stress levels low (American Cancer Society, 2012). By following these screening guidelines and recommendations, both providers and patients are able to take all possible measures to prevent or have early detection of breast cancer.

TEACHING PLAN

This teaching plan offers Advanced Practice Nurses an educational program grounded in review of evidence-based research and guidelines that will assist in providing female patients with screening methods to detect breast cancer and modifiable risk factors that will assist in decreasing the likelihood of disease. The purpose of this teaching plan is to educate Nurse Practitioners' on breast cancer prevention methods for female patients with the goal of increasing Nurse Practitioners' understanding and awareness of breast cancer prevention. This teaching plan will be based on the current standards of practice from the American Cancer Society.

The targeted audience for this presentation is Nurse Practitioners working in primary care centers throughout the community. These nurse practitioners identified with an increased needs assessment for reviewing and furthering their knowledge and understanding of breast cancer prevention in women. Located in Appendix B is the teaching plan for this presentation with outcomes guided by Bloom's Taxonomy. Outcomes of this teaching presentation include that the learner will have an increased understanding and knowledge of breast cancer prevention methods and screenings (cognitive domain), the learner will successfully demonstrate how to conduct a clinical breast exam (psychomotor domain) and the learner will verbalize how the education program will impact further practice with breast cancer prevention in women (affective domain).

Instructional Strategies

Several key methods will be used in providing this teaching presentation to Nurse Practitioners. Direct instructional strategies include the provision of a video demonstration of the correct technique for clinical breast exam provision as well as a lecture review of the current guidelines for breast cancer prevention by the American Cancer Society. Interactive instructional strategies are also used and include practitioner discussion sessions, talking circles and time for peer thought exchange within focus groups.

The direct instructional strategies will focus on providing a presentation of information to the audience through lecture and video centering on screening methods such as breast self-exams, clinical breast exams, mammography, Magnetic Resonance Imaging testing and age related factors in prevention methods. A total of 30 minutes will be allotted for this presentation and review of current practice guidelines. Conversely, 30 minutes of interactive instructional strategies will focus on assessing the level of understanding gained through the presentations and the emotional response of the audience to the information provided. Small groups in talking circles of 4-5 practitioners allow for a sense of privacy and openness in which each practitioner can discuss their response to the teaching program and how it will impact their future practice.

EVALUATION METHODS

Several methods should be used to evaluate the effectiveness of this teaching presentation. A pre-test located in Appendix C should be provided to participants prior to the teaching program to evaluate the knowledge level of practitioners. This pre-test is collected and answers are not discussed with participants at the time. Upon completion of the teaching program, a post-test with the same content as the pre-test should be given to participants. Results of the pre and post-test are compared and participants are able to view their results and determine if their knowledge has improved with the post test.

Success of this teaching presentation will be achieved if learners score a 90% or higher score on the post-test. In addition, at the completion of the teaching program, participants should be provided with an Outcomes Evaluation Form located in Appendix D, in which they will anonymously answer questions regarding their satisfaction with the teaching program and whether it will positively impact their future practice in breast cancer prevention for women.

This educational program was developed with the purpose of providing Advanced Practice Nurses with an educational program for breast cancer prevention in women grounded in review of evidence-based research and guidelines. It is hoped that this presentation will continue to grow and reach a larger number of providers and will most importantly assist Nurse Practitioners in providing female patients with screening methods to detect breast cancer and modifiable risk factors that will assist in decreasing the likelihood of disease.

CONCLUSION

Breast cancer is increasingly becoming a challenge to the global healthcare system. Its burden has been increasing over the past decades. This explains the need for evidence based interventions which can reduce the prevalence and mortality of breast cancer among women.

However, nurse practitioners seem to lack adequate understanding of this disease. Therefore, this teaching plan guides nurse educators on the most appropriate strategies, as well as, providing an opportunity to nurse practitioners to learn the basics of breast cancer management.

References

American Cancer Society. (2012). *Breast Cancer: Early Detection.* Retrieved from http://www.cancer.org/acs/groups/cid/documents/webcontent/003165-pdf.pdf

Barghouti, F. F., Yasein, A., Takruri, A., Hammouri, T., & Qasem, N. (2013). Women's Knowledge and Screening Behaviors regarding Breast Cancer at Family Medicine Clinics. *International Medical Journal, 20*(1), 59-63.

Benard, V. B., Saraiya, M. S., Soman, A., Roland, K. B., Yabroff, K., & Miller, J. (2011). Cancer Screening Practices Among Physicians in the National Breast and Cervical Cancer Early Detection Program. *Journal of Women's Health (15409996), 20*(10), 1479-1484.

Buttaro, T. M., Trybulski, J., Bailey, P. P., & Sandberg-Cook, J. (2013). *Primary Care A Collaborative Practice* (4th ed.). St. Louis, MI: Elsevier Mosby.

Edwards, Q., Maradiegue, A., Seibert, D., Saunders-Goldson, S., & Humphreys, S. (2009). Breast cancer risk elements and nurse practitioners' knowledge, use, and perceived comfort level of breast cancer risk assessment. *Journal of the American Academy of Nurse Practitioners, 21*(5), 270-277.

Edwards, Q., & Seibert, D. (2010). Pre- and posttest evaluation of a breast cancer risk assessment program for nurse practitioners. *Journal of the American Academy of Nurse Practitioners, 22*(7), 376-381.

Fogel, C. I., & Woods, N. F. (2008). *Women's Healthcare in Advanced Practice Nursing.* New York, NY: Springer Publishing Company.

Hart, S., & Bowen, D. (2009). Sexual orientation and intentions to obtain breast cancer screening. *Journal of Women's Health (15409996), 18*(2), 177-185.

Kobetz, E., Menard, J., Barton, B., Maldonado, J., Diem, J., Auguste, P., & Pierre, L. (2010). Barriers to Breast Cancer Screening Among Haitian Immigrant Women in Little Haiti, Miami. *Journal of Immigrant & Minority Health, 12*(4), 520-526.

Mugivhi, N., Maree, J., & Wright, S. (2009). Rural women's knowledge of prevention and care related to breast cancer. *Curationis, 32*(2), 38-45.

Nuño, T., Castle, P. E., Harris, R., Estrada, A., & Team, F. (2011). Breast and Cervical Cancer Screening Utilization Among Hispanic Women Living Near the United States-Mexico Border. *Journal of Women's Health (15409996), 20*(5), 685-693.

Orem, D. E. (1991). *Nursing: Concepts of Practice* (4th ed.). St. Louis, MO: Mosby-Year Book Inc.

Ozanne, E., Wittenberg, E., Garber, J., & Weeks, J. (2010). Breast cancer prevention: patient decision making and risk communication in the high risk setting. *Breast Journal, 16*(1), 38-47.

Ratnasinghe, L., Modali, R., Seddon, M., & Lehman, T. (2010). Physical activity and reduced breast cancer risk: a multinational study. *Nutrition & Cancer, 62*(4), 425-435.

Shalini, Varghese, D., & Nayak, M. (2011). Awareness and Impact of Education on Breast Self Examination Among College Going Girls. *Indian Journal of Palliative Care, 17*(2), 150-154.

Sinicrope, P., Brockman, T., Patten, C., Frost, M., Vierkant, R., Petersen, L., & ... Cerhan, J. (2008). Factors associated with breast cancer prevention communication between mothers and daughters. *Journal of Women's Health (15409996), 17*(6), 1017-1023.

Truesdale-Kennedy, M., Taggart, L., & McIlfatrick, S. (2011). Breast cancer knowledge among women with intellectual disabilities and their experiences of receiving breast mammography. *Journal of Advanced Nursing, 67*(6), 1294-1304.

Watson-Johnson, L. C., DeGroff, A., Steele, C., Revels, M., Smith, J., Justen, E., & ... Richardson, L. C. (2011). Mammography Adherence: A Qualitative Study. *Journal of Women's Health (15409996), 20*(12), 1887-1894.

Yi, M., & Park, E. (2012). Effects of breast health education conducted by trained breast cancer survivors. *Journal of Advanced Nursing, 68*(5), 1100-1110.

Appendix A: Summary of Literature Review Table

Summary of Review of Literature						
Study	Design	Methods	Sample	Tools	Findings	Limitations
1 Edwards & Seibert (2010)	QN	Outcome Analysis, Pre-test Post-test design	35 NPs at a national NP conference	Breast Cancer Risk Assessment (BrCRA) education program developed by researchers	Continuing education through the implementation of a BrCRA program significantly increased NPs knowledge in assessing breast cancer risk.	Convenience sampling that prevents generalizability of the findings to all NPs
2 Yi and Park (2011)	QN	Pre and Post Test, quasi-experimental design	22 young healthy Korean women ages 20-40	60 minute education program developed by researchers consisting of 2 components: breast cancer general knowledge and how to practice breast self-exam	A one-time breast health class can be useful in motivating young women to adopt behaviors that help to prevent breast cancer morbidity and mortality	Study was conducted in Korea – generalizability of the results to other women from other geographical areas or countries may be limited. Small sample
3 Edwards et al. (2009)	QN	Descriptive Study	Convenience sample of 147 NPs attending a national NP conference	Survey developed by the researchers to obtain specific knowledge of breast cancer risk assessment	Assessing women's risk for the development of breast cancer is important in providing primary and secondary preventative strategies	Small convenience sample size of 147 NPs- 5 % of total conference attendees
4 Bernard et al. (2011)	QN	Descriptive Study, split sample design	A nationally represented sample of 1,111 primary care physicians from the AMA's physician master file	Survey and questionnaire developed by researchers with specific outcome measures	Beliefs and screening practices for breast cancer are similar between physician members of the NBCCEDP and non-program providers	Observations may have been influenced by specialty. Limited sample size
5 Shalini, Varghese & Nayak (2011)	QN	Experimental design, pre-test post-test design	40 female students between ages	3 part questionnaire:	72% of participants had average knowledge on BSE.	Study limited to only 40 female

15

			18-19 from selected colleges in the district of Udupi	Demographics, BSE knowledge assessment and teaching program	Only 1 student was performing BSE occasionally	students from only 1 district
6 Ozanne et al. (2010)	QL	Survey Study	146 high risk patients in breast cancer diagnosis interviewed by 4 physicians	Patient interviews and patient questionnaires	Women at high risk for breast cancer face challenging decisions and difficulty in comprehending information	The data wa collected at jus one setting. Patients wer interviewed b only physicians, small grou from which it i difficult to dra conclusions about population
7 Johnson et al.(2011)	QL	Exploratory Study, focus group methodology	128 women in 20 focus group across 5 cities in the US. Sample includes White, Hispanic, Japanese-American, Blacks.	Focus groups discussions moderated by a facilitator segmented by age, insurance status and self-identification of ethnicity	Five barriers to routine mammography screening: concerns about test efficacy, personal concerns about procedure, access to mammography, psychosocial issues and cultural factors	Study resul may not b generalized beyond th women studie due to nature e study bei focus group
8 Ratnasinghe et al. (2009)	QN	Epidemiologic, multinational study	1,463 breast cancer cases and 4,862 controls	Questionnaire where subjects were asked how many times and how long they exercise	Physical activity may reduce breast cancer risk regardless of race, weight, or family history of breast cancer	Recall bias ar selection bi could hav influenced results.
9 Hart & Bowen (2009)	QN	Longitudinal study	150 self-identified bisexual/lesbian women and 400 heterosexual women	Questionnaires about breast cancer screening attitudes at baseline and at a 6 month follow-up	Attitudes and beliefs about breast cancer screenings and medical providers impact lesbian/bisexual women's willingness to plan for mammography	Samples we self-selected which may lim generalizabilit of finding Samples we also compris of women w are interest in breast cand risk.

10 Barghouti et al. (2013)	QN	Cross-sectional study	602 female patients aged 20 years and above	Self-administered questionnaire with researcher questions	Being married and having a good knowledge score predict more BSE practice	¼ of the sample was reluctant to apply the screening methods to due fatalistic beliefs.
11 Kobetz et al. (2010)	QL	Grounded theory	15 out of a random selection of 300 Haitian immigrant women who had participated in a previous research initiative	Interview with open ended questions and questionnaires	3 barriers to breast cancer screening : structural, psychosocial and socio-cultural	The final sample number of 15 is too small to make generalizations about the women in Little Haiti as a whole
12 Nuno et al. (2011)	QN	Randomized control trial / Cross-sectional study	504 women aged 50 and above residing in Yuma County, Arizona	Survey instrument developed from researchers and community stake holders.	Women who received a recommendation to get a mammogram and pap smear from a clinician were more likely to do so within 1 year	Because the questionnaires were interviewer administered, social desirability may have biased some responses
13 Kennedy, Taggart & McIlfatrick (2010)	QN	Descriptive study, focus group methodology	19 women identified as having a borderline to moderate intellectual disability	4 focus groups with semi-structured interviews developed from the literature and research team's personal experience	A lack of information and embarrassment was identified as the main barriers to screening for this group	Small sample size of this study affects transferability of findings
14 Sinicrope et al. (2008)	QN and QL	Open-ended question analysis, Generalized estimating equation methodology	1778 women from 355 families across Minnesota	Questionnaires where women were asked whether or not they had provided advice to their daughters on breast cancer prevention methods	Breast cancer prevention behaviors were associated with provision of advice from mothers to daughters	Only mothers were surveyed, not daughters.
15 Mugivhi, Maree & Wright (2009)	QL	Exploratory and contextual study	200 women living in a rural province	Structured interviews to participants	Women were unable to take responsibility for their breast health due to lack of knowledge	Convenient sampling. Data gathered was self-reported

							and subject recall bias.
Summary	10 QN, 4 QL, 1 both QN and QL	QN mostly descriptive as well as pre and post test analysis. Also 1 longitudinal study and 2 cross-sectional studies. QL mostly exploratory with 1 grounded theory and 1 survey phenomenological study.	Sample size ranged from 15 to 1778. All participants were women ages 18 and above with most over 40. Most were based in communities throughout the country.	QL studies mostly used subject interviews and questionnaires. QN studies mostly used researcher developed surveys and questionnaires. Some QN studies used education programs including the BrCRA.	The level of knowledge, attitude and understanding of breast cancer risks as well as prevention methods were found to be major factors that either prevented or assisted women in seeking care for breast cancer prevention. Medical providers also play an important role in breast cancer prevention.	Multiple studi had sm sample size Selection a self-reported, subject rec bias also fou to be limiti generalizabili of findings.

Appendix B: Teaching Plan Outline

Title of Offering:	Teaching Plan on breast cancer prevention in women for Nurse Practitioners						
Purpose:	To educate Nurse Practitioners on breast cancer prevention methods for female patients						
Goal:	To increase Nurse Practitioners' understanding and awareness of breast cancer preventi						
Target Audience:	☑ ARNP's ☐ Patients ☐ Staff			Contact Hours:	60 minutes	Total Clock Hours:	60 min

Learner Objectives	Content Outline	Method of Presentation	Time Allotted	Resources	Method of Evaluation	Outcom
1) The learner will have an increased understanding and knowledge of breast cancer prevention methods and screenings (cognitive domain)	1.1 Provide American Cancer Society (ACS) Guidelines for breast cancer screening	1.Presentation of ACS guidelines to learners	15 minutes	American Cancer Society breast cancer prevention screenings for providers	Pre-test, Post-test	Learners achieve a score or 9 the post tes

2) The learner will successfully demonstrate how to conduct a clinical breast exam (psychomotor domain)	2.1 Showcasing of clinical breast exam by a provider	2. Video showcasing adequate demonstration of clinical breast exam by a provider	15 minutes	Video on clinical breast exams and live breast models	Return demonstration on provided breast models	Learner will successfully demonstrate clinical breast exam on breast models
3) the learner will verbalize how the education program will impact further practice with breast cancer prevention in women (affective domain)	3.1 Discussion and talking circles among learners concerning emotional response and impact that education program will provide in future practice.	3.1 Small group format of 4-5 nurse practitioners with one practitioner as group spokesperson 3.2 spokespersons to provide report to the whole class of impact of teaching plan on group members	15 minutes of small group discussion 15 minute presentation of discussion findings from group spokesperson to whole class	Notepads, pens, discussion questions	Group spokesperson's report of what impact teaching plan will have on future practice of group members	Learner will identify and describe positive impact this teaching program will have on breast cancer prevention care to female patients
References:	American Cancer Society. (2012). Breast cancer: Early detection. Retrieved from http://www.cancer.org/acs/groups/cid/documents/webcontent/003165-pdf.pdf					

Breast Cancer Prevention in Women

Pre-Test and Post-Test for Nurse Practitioners

1. What is the recommended age by the American Cancer Society for women to begin mammography testing?

   A. 30 years

   B. 35 years

   C. 40 years

   D. 45 years

2. How often should a clinical breast exam be conducted?

   A. Yearly

   B. Weekly

   C. Bi-Annually

   D. Every other year

3. How often should a breast self-exam be conducted?

   A. Every other month before menstruation

   B. Every 3 months after menstruation

   C. Every month 3-4 days after menstruation

   D. Every month 3-4 days before menstruation

4. What are modifiable risk factors for breast cancer?

   A. Maintaining a healthy weight

   B. Moderate cardiovascular exercise 3-4 times a week

   C. Maintaining a healthy diet

   D. Smoking cessation

   E. All of the above

5. What is the Brevagen test?

    A. A screening test that assist in staging breast cancer

    B. A diagnostic test that determines at what age breast cancer will be diagnosed

    C. A diagnostic test that confirms breast cancer diagnosis

    D. A screening test that assist providers in determining lifetime and 5 year percentage risk of developing breast cancer

6. Who should have the Brevagen test?

    A. All women beginning age 35

    B. All women beginning age 40

    C. All women beginning age 55

    D. All women beginning age 45

7. What is BrCA testing?

    A. A screening test for breast cancer percentage risk in women with a high risk of breast cancer from a first degree relative

    B. A diagnostic test for breast cancer diagnosis

    C. A diagnostic test that assist in staging breast cancer

    D. A screening test for breast cancer in children

8. At what age should BrCA testing be conducted?

    A. Age 30 with a first degree relative with breast cancer

    B. Age 50 with a first degree relative with breast cancer

    C. Age 35 with a first degree relative with breast cancer

    D. At any age for women who have a first degree relative with breast cancer

9. True or False:

    Level of alcohol consumption has been linked to the development of breast cancer

10. True or False:

Medical providers including nurse practitioners are at the forefront of breast health education and breast cancer prevention in women.

Answers:

1. C
2. A
3. C
4. E
5. D
6. A
7. A
8. D
9. True
10. Tue

Appendix D: Outcomes Achievement Evaluation Form

Outcomes Evaluation Form for Teaching Plan Participants

1. After this teaching presentation, has your knowledge of breast cancer prevention screenings increased?

   A. Yes

   B. No

   C. There is no change in my knowledge

2. Has your comfort level in performing breast exam increased after this presentation?

   A. Yes

   B. No

   C. There is no change in my comfort level

3. Will this education program positively impact your future practice for breast cancer prevention in women?
   A. Yes
   B. No
   C. There is no impact to my future practice

4. How likely are you to participate in continuing education regarding breast cancer prevention in women as a practitioner?
   A. Very likely
   B. Likely
   C. Unlikely
   D. Very unlikely
   E. There will be no change from my current level of continuing education

5. Overall, has this teaching plan assisted you in becoming a better provider with increased comfort and knowledge regarding breast cancer prevention?
   A. Yes
   B. No
   C. There is no change

6. How likely are you to recommend this course and this instructor to a colleague?
   A. Very likely
   B. Likely
   C. Unlikely
   D. Very unlikely

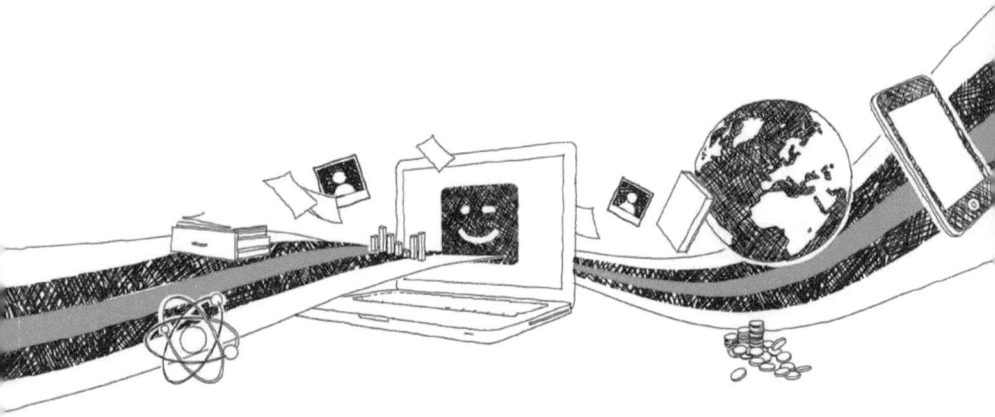
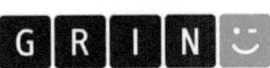